Praise for Fresh Off the Couch!

"Fresh Off the Couch is a must read for anyone new to or returning to fitness training. Cris and Marla capture the essence of connecting with lifetime fitness."

~Sally Edwards
The Head Heart, Heart Zones™ USA
TREK Women's Triathalon Spokeswoman

"Finally a book that's all about me! This individualized plan for lifelong fitness is easy to understand, empowering and effective without guilt, judgment or spandex!"

~Heidi Shepherd, M.Ed.
Faculty, Social and Human Services,
Lake Washington Technical College

"Bravo to Cris and Marla for helping others 'get off the couch' and to finding the fun in fitness while giving them the skills to maintain it for a lifetime."

~Cheryl Marek
Personal Trainer
world record holder in endurance cycling

"A fresh look at fitness that will make you laugh, make you smarter, AND get you moving! Fresh Off the Couch is an easy to read, user friendly guide to sustainable fitness. This book empowers people to take control of their body image, set appropriate goals, and focus their fitness in all realms: mental, emotional, and physical."

~Deb Chickadel
Educator

"If you're sick and tired of feeling bad about your seeming inability to get, this is the book for you. Presenting information in a humorous way, the authors put our attention squarely where it should be: on our own physical health and well-being. This book crashes through the guilt and bad feelings and helps you realize that every effort toward becoming healthier is meaningful and worthwhile. Interesting facts throughout the book are often surprising and provide even more motivation to get "Fresh Off the Couch!"

~Julianna Ross
Working Mom

"Inside these pages, you'll find inspiration for a life made better through movement of the mind and body. Using language we can all understand, Fresh Off the Couch explains why we don't exercise and offers tools to help us get out there and try. Wake up to a modern view of what it means to be fit!"

~Ruth Sved
Avid reader and believer in mind-body connection

"This is an excellent book especially for those who have difficulty getting started on the road to better health. So many people can't get started getting fit because they don't know what to do and so many people quit because they are aiming at the wrong targets. Fresh Off the Couch, helps focus us on what our goals should be – fitness, not thinness. The authors have done a great job laying out a comprehensive approach to getting fit. This book discusses many of the problems that get in our way on the way to better health."

~Dr. Eugene Kearney
Chiropractic Physician and marathon runner

"*Fresh Off the Couch is the perfect support for those beginning a new journey with their bodies! I love the perspective about fitness. In a culture where image, distortions about body size and shape leave people feeling hopeless about having a real relationship with food and movement this book gives an easy to follow plan that leads to fitness and fun!*"

~LeAnn Gibbs
Author of *The Divine Cowgirls Guide to Fully Living*

"*This fun and fact filled book makes it easy for anyone to Get Off the Couch and onto the road of lifelong fitness. It arms the reader with the most recent research. Using humor, the authors challenge our former ideas on size and fitness and give step-by-step plans on how to finally make it into the ranks of the fit. I recommend this book to all my patients!*

~Carla Corrado, PT, LMP
Faculty, Cornish College of the Arts
Kinesiology, Conditioning and Movement Foundations

"*A new approach: nice, simple and straightforward. This book shows beginners why they don't have to be an Ironman™ to be fit and teaches them how to use a heart rate monitor to get in touch with their own body. A great first book!*"

~Carl Foster, Ph.D.

Fresh Off the Couch!

*"What You Didn't Know About Fitness
Makes All the Difference"*

Marla Fields and Cris Kessler

B&H Bennett &
Hastings Publishing

Cover design and graphics by Kirsten Adams
Illustration by Kirsten Adams.
kirstenadams.com

For more information or to reach the authors visit:
www.freshoffthecouch.com

ISBN 978-1-934733-33-2
paperback, 112 pages

B&H Bennett &
Hastings Publishing

Contents

Introduction

Newton's first law of Motion, sometimes referred to as the Law of Inertia, does not involve apples. It involves bodies, bodies who are moving and bodies who are not moving.

So what does Newton's first law of Motion tell us?

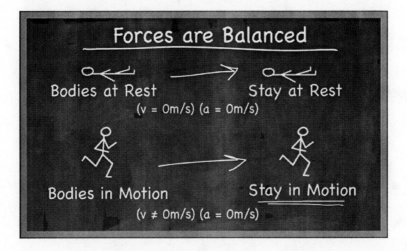

- *If all things are balanced, a body that is at rest stays at rest.*

- *And if a body is in motion, it stays in motion.*

What does that mean to some one who wants to get fit?

It means it's a scientific fact that there are forces out there working to keep you at rest.

The forces keeping you on the couch include:

- inertia
- gravity
- fear of failure
- the remote control

This book was designed to counteract these forces with a new kind of fitness plan, using psychological techniques sprinkled with a dash of humor to help get a body off the couch and in motion. The slow building, consistent type, that keeps a body in motion. That is the way to get fit and stay fit!

Begin Where You Are

Where Else Would You Start?

Fitness is a language many don't speak. When you are "Fresh off the Couch" the fitness world can seem like a foreign land filled with sports nuts who bike to work and overenthusiastic friends who want to sign you up to do a triathlon, a half marathon or an Ironman™. "It's easy and fun," they keep harping year after year. The problem is that for most people outside of the fitness world, "Iron Man" is a movie based on a Marvel comic character.

Then they explain: being an Ironman™ means you can, swim 2.4 miles, bike 112 miles and run 26.2 miles: all in one day!

People who are "into" fitness may seem like they are in a world of their own.... You, like most people, may think that world is a place you want to go. You may have even been there, but after a few attempts you have returned to the couch. It seems worth trying to adapt to that world, but it just gets harder and harder to even begin.

Now you are planning another venture into that fabulous fitness world... This time be aware that there is a force at work against you. It is the law of inertia, and it has some powerful allies in popular culture (not to mention the furniture section). This time you will not go alone. This book is designed to help you overcome those forces. It is your guide into the world of fitness.

How to Use this Book

The first thing we're going to do is equip your mind with *Radical Ideas* and *Power Buttons*: quick tips and short quips you can memorize and pull out in a handy fashion. We've marked them with icons to make them easy to spot.

 Radical Ideas: This icon marks an idea that probably will shake up some of your existing beliefs about fitness.

 Power Buttons: This icon marks an empowering thought or action you can adopt.

This book is packed with *Radical Ideas* and *Power Buttons* to help you make changes in your life. They are designed to ease the transition into the mind-set of fitness; much like a phrase book eases the transition when visiting a foreign country.

Each chapter in this book starts with an explanation of ideas and concepts, followed by a plan to help you put the ideas into practice. Each ends with a do-able exercise plan that will help you practice the ideas in that chapter.

Read each chapter, but don't begin the exercises in them until you've reached the day of the week that lists them in the exercise plan. These exercise plans (which involve sometimes mental and sometimes physical exercises) will expand your awareness of the fitness choices you make. As you become aware of your fitness choices, you will actually be strengthening your ability to choose. You will be gaining awareness of your choices while increasing your fitness level.

 Following the weekly exercise plans (consisting of both mental and physical exercises) will bring you more freedom through awareness.

Improving your fitness level will improve your health, your self-esteem and your life.

Good News:
Things Have Changed in
the World of Fitness!

And what we didn't know about fitness makes all the difference!

Over the last decade studies have changed what scientists know about health and fitness, and what they know is astonishingly different from what most people believe is true. This new information means living a fit lifestyle and being a healthy, fit person becomes an attainable goal for everyone, regardless of body type.

There is a growing library of research challenging the myths and assumptions we have collectively made about fitness and weight for decades[1]*. This book is an addition to that library, but this book is different. (We know... you've heard that before, but this book really is different! !) It is a guide that will teach you to

---

* Notes are at the end of each chapter.

apply the new fitness research in a way that will remain with you.

More importantly, fitness is different!

 Fitness is achievable for everyone because some of the rules of fitness have changed.

Size is not the issue when it comes to health. Fitness is the issue. That simple statement sets the stage for a new era of fitness.

This book will teach you how to take your focus off weight and put it on fitness, where it belongs. We will map out the journey in small, doable steps.

Let's begin right where you are, today. You don't have to change or do anything before you start. Just reading this book with an open mind is enough to begin on the road to fitness.

So... Where Are You?

To find your starting point let's take a closer look at what you think right now about fitness and yourself.

◈ Does the force of gravity seem stronger when you are around your couch?

◈ Do you walk a flight of stairs easily or do you huff and puff?

◈ Does your ideal weight come from a height/weight chart?

◈ Do you spend more time thinking about fitness than you do participating in fitness activities?

◈ Do you have a reliable way of measuring what it means to be unfit or fit?

Best Kept Secrets about Body Weight and Health

Where did you first learn how much you should weigh? Many people learned from a height/weight chart that was frequently referenced by physicians, parents and popular magazines: this infamous chart was created in the 1940's by the Metropolitan Life Insurance Company, and it erroneously correlated weight with life expectancy.

 Many authorities based our past ideals of fitness on a weight chart that was not scientifically produced.

A more recent, popular measurement tool has been Body Mass Index (BMI). To calculate a person's BMI divide their weight by the square of their height and then multiply that figure by 703[2]. The BMI measurement was developed somewhere in the mid 1800s by a Belgian mathematician and statistician named Lambert Adolphe Quatelet[3]. Quatelet was one of the first scientists to mix mathematics and statistics with the social sciences. He developed the BMI to provide statistical data about the height and weight ratio of people from different geographical areas.

15

It is important to know that the BMI was created as a way for scientists to describe body types of a population. It is not an accurate measure of anything for an individual. BMI was designed to describe the appearance of a group or a population. It certainly cannot gauge a person's health in any meaningful way.

Now take a deep breath and savor for a moment what you have just learned and what it really means.... *You can be healthy, live as long as genetically possible and not constantly worry about the ideal height-weight chart or the BMI!* As surprising as it might seem, this is the new world of health sciences: **how fit you are has little to do with what you weigh.**

Just consider for a moment a world where fitness has not much to do with your pants size, large or small. This is "good" news because it takes the focus off weight. So take note: if you are considered by the culture to be the "right" weight you will still have to actually do activities to increase your fitness.

 Weight loss does not by itself increase fitness.

Unfortunately for most people in the American culture, fitness is thought to be exclusively determined by how much body fat you do or don't have. If you are slim, chances are that people (including your doctor) have a bias that you are fit. And the reverse is true as well. If you are heavier, people probably assume you are unfit. Both assumptions are wrong: you can be thin and unfit, or fat and unfit, or any weight in between and unfit.

For some people this new information is scary. Right away they think it will lead to uncontrollable behavior, like running barefoot through all-you-can-eat buffets. We believe this information will lead people to focus on what is really important: mental and physical fitness. (So if you do run into the occasional all-you-can-eat buffet, you will finally be able to enjoy yourself!)

We know now that the old ideas are harmful; doing people of all sizes a disservice. An article in the May 2007 American Journal of Public Health disagreed with the National Institute of Health's practice of applying the label "overweight" to older women in the BMI category 25 to 29.9, because women in that range actually had the lowest mortality rate

Based on the old ideas, people are drawing the wrong conclusions about their health and the health of their children, loved ones, clients or patients. Too many health professionals treat thin people like they are fit and anyone with a BMI over 25 like they are unfit, neglecting to measure that individual's actual fitness indicators.

 Body fat, height and weight are relatively easy to measure; but they are not good measures of health and fitness.

Earlier we asked you questions about your thoughts and beliefs regarding your personal fitness. Maybe some of these have already changed. If you were basing your fitness evaluation on height-to-weight ratios or BMI, you need a way to get a better fix on your own personal fitness. By looking at your own levels of strength, flexibility and endurance, the first week of exercises are going to help you correctly evaluate where you are right now.

The Power of Choice

We will now introduce ideas associated with Choice Theory[4]. Working with these will help you take stock of where you are now, mentally and physically. Some Choice Theory ideas that apply are:

1. It is in your power to feel better about yourself and the world around you.

2. To develop this power takes practice.

3. Outside influences cannot force you to feel, act or think in a predetermined way.

The process of accepting our present fitness and our future health can be daunting at first but take heart, there is hope.

 Wherever you are now, be assured that you got there under your own power.

18

You don't believe it was your choice to end up on the couch?

You don't believe you would choose to be unfit?

Maybe it feels that way.

The inspirational life of actor Christopher Reeves presents examples of the power of choice.

One day he was "Superman" and the next day he was unable to move his body. If you are thinking that becoming dependent on a wheelchair was not his choice, you are right. The relevant choice came after the accident. Consider the choices Mr. Reeves had after his accident confined him to a wheelchair and a respirator: he could give up, or he could move forward.

The idea that outside influences cannot force you to feel, act, or think in a certain way means recognizing your own power. That is the mindset that allowed Mr. Reeves to move forward.

 You have gotten where you are under your own power. Understanding allows you to move forward with that same power.

The reason Mr. Reeves was an inspiration to so many was that after the accident he decided to live his life as fully as he could. One might even say his fame grew greater *after* the accident. Although this is a very

19

extreme example, the principle is the same for everyone. Everyone faces those same two choices every minute of every day, you can give up or move forward.

Hopefully most of your choices will not be under such extreme circumstances.

Regardless of the situation, the first thing is to accept all the power you actually have, not over others, but the power to choose what you want for yourself.

 You choose. You are the only one in charge of yourself and your decisions.

It's one thing to realize you make all the choices for yourself; it's a bit trickier figuring out what choices to make once you recognize you have all this freedom to choose. You have already decided to visit the world of fitness, and you're going to get there under your own power.

But before we start, we need to think about what it means and looks like to be fit.

Who Sets the Standard for Your Fitness?

For many people, media sources like magazines and MTV set the standard for beauty and fitness. Elevating those images to the level of "model" will lead to wrong conclusions about the true nature and culture of fitness.

Let's look at how this plays out in real life:

◇ Did you know that many professional athletes have height/weight ratios that would place them in the ranks of the morbidly obese?

 Fitness cannot really be measured by size. Better measures would be strength, endurance and flexibility.

◇ Did you know that a veteran costumer for film and MTV shared that many singers, especially female singers, can't even sit down in the clothes they wear in music videos? They are wearing costumes designed to appeal to our fantasies, and they are so tight they can only be worn while standing!

This example shows how ridiculous it is to base our ideas of fitness on images designed to appeal to our fantasies. Take a few seconds to look into your own ideas about the world of fitness: if there is an MTV costume there, please let out the seams! As we saw above, even professional athletes often outweigh the traditional height/weight charts. Think about how ironic it is if you, even subconsciously, are connecting your idea of fitness to something that wasn't even designed to fit!

The influence of media is so pervasive that most people do not know that fitness is not determined by size. What with the distractions of fitness fantasies and misguided measurements, valid fitness indicators **strength, flexibility** and **endurance** are often overlooked. It's not the size or weight of a person, it's the qualities of their body that determine fitness.

 You are okay at the size you are right now.

People's reactions to this idea vary. It is freeing to a former football star who is now a utility company lineman. He weighs 300 pounds, but he easily climbs up and down many telephone poles each day, lugging with him several pounds of equipment. He no longer spends energy listening to people who say he needs to lose weight. To a few people, it has been bittersweet. One young woman was devastated when she finally understood she was okay at her current size. She said it was upsetting for her to realize that she had wasted years of her life wishing she was a different size and trying to change her body type.

It is difficult to filter out cultural expectations when forming a picture of what is healthy. Something that is often overlooked is the fact that genetics play a significant role in body type and size. What does this mean? Thinking about the impact of genetics on body type and size can be more easily understood if we set aside the human element. The young woman mentioned above would have been less distressed about her size if she had been able to look at body types through a different lens: that of man's best friend.

Body Types: What Kind of Dog Are You?

Dogs are a fun way to think about natural body types when considering "where you are" physically.

They come in a huge variety, based on their genes, just like people. In fact, there are an almost infinite number of dog types, almost as many as people types.

In this week's exercises we'll be asking you, "What kind of dog are you?" Or rather, if you were a dog, what kind would be most like your physical type? Okay...maybe you're not that hairy and you don't slobber, but you get the idea.

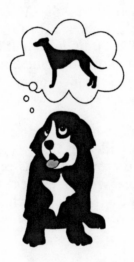

It makes for a tough life if you are a St. Bernard or a Newfoundland spending your life wishing you were shaped like a Greyhound or a Whippet.

What if you are just perfect for a Newfoundland? What would be wrong with that?

Do you think when a Chihuahua looks at a Newfoundland she's thinking, "Look at that big fat dog!"?

In the dog world, it's the American Kennel Club (AKC) that sets the standard for fitness and perfection, and it is a fact that an underweight St. Bernard would never win Best in Show. Imagine having the genes of a Newfoundland and trying to starve and exercise a body down to look like a Whippet!

Genetically most of us would not qualify as AKC purebreds, so our ideal genetic type will be based on a mixture of inputs. As part of the evaluation in this week's exercises we are asking you to take a look at your family photos to get an idea of what is splashing around in your gene pool.

Let's say you are ready to start where you are. You now have an idea where you are starting from, and you know that your ideal has nothing to do with cultural icons but is based on your genetics. You know that fitness is not about size, but is about strength, endurance and flexibility. You know that you have the power to make choices; that you have gotten where you are under your own power and that using the same power you can move forward to fitness, depending on what you choose. So how do you make choices that help you become more fit?

We've been talking about fitness as journey, but rather than focusing on the features of the journey, we'd like you to focus on fitness behaviors. Fitness behavior is made up of a set of habits. Habits that are much like brushing your teeth.

Your dental routines are good habits to consider when building a path for fitness behaviors. There are many similarities: If your goal is "perfect dental health" you can run into many of the same pitfalls as you do if "perfect health and fitness" is your goal. Genes determine much of your dental health, as they do body type. Daily brushing and flossing are invaluable to maintaining good dental health, and for physical fitness, exercise should be an *almost* daily affair. (We'll talk more about that.) Fitness, like having clean teeth, is a choice.

We stated above that for physical fitness, exercise should be an *almost* daily affair. This comes as a surprise to many people because there is a prevailing idea that you must work out, all out, as often as you can, in order to get fit. This idea is wrong and leads to injuries and discouragement, which is the path that runs directly back to the couch.

 Rest is critical to successful fitness goals.

"So," you might be thinking, "what comes next?"

25

The answer is simple; follow the exercises on the chart for this chapter. They are designed to help increase your awareness and have you focus on your fitness at the same time. Each exercise plan is designed to start you on the principles of working out smarter so that you can achieve your goals faster. With this chapter, the focus is on showing that it's important to accept and love your starting point... or at least just accept it for now.

The ideas in this book are simple, but require practice.

 It takes practice for changes to stick. Remember that practice is just that: it's practice not perfection.

Exercise Plan

This week's plan will help you assess where you are right now. You find out how much time you really have in a week and help you determine what's in your gene pool. We encourage you to do all the steps in these plans because each is designed to develop both your mental and physical muscles toward sustainable fitness.

	"BEGIN WHERE YOU ARE" WORKOUT CHART
Day 1	• Look at your people. Find out what your parents and grandparents looked like at your age. Find pictures if you can and keep in a folder for Day Two. • If information about your biological family is not available, look in the mirror. Do you think your genetic heritage would make you more attune with a Labrador or a Chihuahua? **Do not do any additional exercise today.**
Day 2	• What "type" of dog are you? Pick a breed that most suits your family's body type. Write down the name of this breed and at least three traits that you most like about this type of dog. **Do not do any additional exercise today.**
Day 3	• Fill in the "How Much Time Do You Have" Chart on the next page. **Do not do any additional exercise today.**
Day 4	**REST DAY** **Do not do any exercise today.**
Day 5	• Take stock of your physical body. List 3 activities you can do and like to do. **Do not do any additional exercise today.**
Day 6	• Write down your daily routine for maintaining your dental health. Write down what makes it easy or hard to complete your daily dental health routine. • Write down your current daily fitness routine. It is okay if you are starting with no current fitness routine, after all, this book is for those "Fresh Off the Couch." **Do not do any additional exercise today.**
Day 7	• Are you ready to make a change*? If yes, then list three reasons. If you are not ready to make a change put this book down immediately! *Warning: this book could lead to change! **Do not do any additional exercise today.**

27

HOW MUCH TIME DO YOU REALLY HAVE IN A WEEK?

	DAILY TOTALS	WEEKLY TOTALS
How many hours do you sleep per night?		
How much time do you need for meals per day?		
How many hours do you work per day? (Add in commute.)		
How many hours do you go to school per day (includes carpooling kids, etc.)?		
How much time do you need right now for daily care? (Shower, getting dressed, brushing teeth, exercise.)		
GRAND TOTAL (add all columns up and put totals here.) Multiply daily totals x 7 to get weekly totals.		
Total Hours in a week:	**168**	
Subtract your grand weekly total:	-	
Which leaves you with your free hours in a single week:	————	

Chapter Endnotes

[1] Books like *Rethinking Thin: The New Science of Weight Loss* by *New York Times* science writer Gina Kolata, *The Obesity Myth: Why America's Obsession with Weight is Hazardous to Your Health* by Paul Campos and *Big Fat Lies: The Truth about Your Weight and Your Health* by Glenn A. Gaesser, Ph.D. are just a few that challenge the fifty billion dollar a year diet and exercise industry with new scientific information.

[2] A person 5'6" and 155 lbs. or a person 5'11" and 179 lbs would have a 25 BMI.

[3] It was then called the Quatelet Index.

[4] Choice Theory is a method of looking at choices, developed by Dr. William Glasser of the Glasser Institute.

Nibbling Around the Edge
Food for Thought

The chart below describes four people with varying fitness and fatness levels. Look at the chart and answer this question: which of the people described below dies first?

FIT & LEAN	FIT & FAT
UNFIT & LEAN	UNFIT & FAT

Let's look to Dr. Stephen N. Blair of the University of South Carolina and the Cooper Institute for the answer[5].

Dr. Blair's research shows that unfit people at *any* size die first. Fit people at *any* weight live longer than unfit people. So that means fitness—not fatness—predicts a longer life. Statistically, fit people of all sizes die at the same rate, regardless of size or fat.

 Fat is not the issue, fitness is.

We are finding out it isn't better to be thin at any cost. In fact thin isn't the point at all. Our bodies are smart. We know this because our ancestors would have never been able to reproduce and raise offspring if their bodies had been unable store extra food when they were lucky enough to get it. Smart bodies burn up calories only when they are needed. In fact it would make no sense from a survival point of view if gaining weight and storing fat hurt your health.

Recently, there is a lot of media coverage on the claim that there is an "obesity" epidemic. But the media has been highlighting only part of the story.

After looking at the studies themselves, and not the sensationalized headlines, a different picture emerges... Physical activity or lack of physical activity in daily life is the real key to health.

Scientific studies such as the ones entitled, "Fitness Level, Not Body Fat, May be a Stronger Indicator of Longevity in Older Adults"[6] and "Associations between Body Composition, Anthropometry and Mortality in Women aged 65 years and older"[7] show that women with the lowest mortality rate had a BMI of 25 to 30. (Remember that describes a person approximately 5'6" and 155 lbs to 186 lbs.)

These are two of the new studies that back up the radical idea that fitness is the issue—not weight.

Although this is definitely a radical idea, the response does not need to be radical. In fact some of these same studies show that longevity can be increased by a relatively light to moderate amount of exercise.

We have all heard the saying "Eat to live, don't live to eat." Fitness is like that as well. Too often people are slaves to fitness and eating regimes that are designed around a fear of fat.

Exercise Is Not a Punishment for Being Fat or Unfit

 The key is to eat well and train to be healthy so that you can live a free, fun and happy life. Fitness training and eating well should be used as a tool, not as bludgeoning instrument.

To help clarify this Power Button let's look at the dictionary definition of health:[8]

1a: the condition of being sound in body, mind, or spirit; *especially*: freedom from physical disease or pain **b:** the general condition of the body <enjoys good *health*>

2a: flourishing condition: **WELL-Being b:** general condition or state.

Ask yourself: What would it take for me to **flourish**, to have a sound body, mind and spirit?

Unfortunately the old insurance industry height/weight charts and BMI have too often been the accepted measurement for health, but they don't measure health. Health measured by size is woefully inadequate.

 Size may be an indicator of a problem, but size is <u>not</u> the problem.

Here is a good example: When one of the authors of this book was pregnant with her first child, the Ob/Gyn doctor, a petite woman, was a bit concerned by the unborn child's head size. She was so concerned in fact that she emailed the sonograms to a specialist. When asked why this particular specialist was being consulted, the answer was that the baby's head measurement was unusually large: there could be a chance that the baby had hydrocephalus (water on the brain). In the office with the Ob/Gyn and the specialist on speakerphone, the parents sat down for a very serious meeting. The Ob/Gyn explained in detail her fears about the baby's gigantic head size. After what seemed like forever the Ob/Gyn gave the specialist a chance to speak... After a thoughtful sigh, the specialist asked, "Do the parent's have large heads?" The Ob/Gyn slowly looked up at the parents' St. Bernard size heads. It was priceless to see the realization slowly hit her. That's right, not everyone is a tiny little Chihuahua with a tiny Chihuahua size head.

When health is measured with the BMI and height/weight charts, it oversimplifies the questions and the answers. It gives people a false sense of control over their health by providing a simple solution: change your weight. The problem with this very simple solution is that losing weight does not improve your health. In fact, research shows that dieting, especially the gaining/losing/gaining type of dieting can have serious health consequences.

Many people are now realizing that the arbitrary definition of *obesity* means that many very *fit* and *healthy* people are now considered *obese*. It is easy to see that there are many genetic types that allow an individual to carry weight and be fit. What is also true is that there are many genetic types that allow individuals to be skinny and remain unfit and unhealthy.

On the other hand health, flexibility, strength and endurance are not easily measured and tend to naturally fluctuate around life's experiences. And being fit is not a destination, it is a process.

For the purposes of this book we need to separate what is fit and healthy from what is a social expectation.

For you to get what you want, you need to know what you want.

Choice #1: To be as healthy and fit as you can be.

If you picked this choice, congratulations! You have picked a choice you can achieve, live happily and have fun with!

Here is how to do this: You need moderate exercise approximately 20–30 minutes per day, five to six times per week. New ways to use a heart rate monitor will make exercising more efficient by incorporating biofeedback into your workout. (We will show you how in the chapter, "Using your Heart to Change Your Mind About Fitness.") You also need to eat healthy, whole and satisfying food. You need to eat enough healthy oils, fruits and vegetables, and fiber each day. Adding fruits, vegetables and fiber to the recommended amounts per day is a good way to have a healthier diet.

Back to the dog analogy: If you have a healthy and fit dog you need to give her enough water and good food. You can't have a healthy pet if you just feed her treats. But you can't really have a happy dog if she never gets any treats either. Also your dog needs the proper amount of exercise for the breed. A general rule for dogs is the same for people: 20–30 minutes of walking per day. You just can't walk the dog for two hours, one day a week and expect the dog to be okay. The dog would be better off if you split up the walking time over the whole week and so will you.

We are not really comparing people to dogs, but it may be easier to visualize basic needs when it comes to pet health. This way you can see the basic needs without the added complications of being human. A pet needs basic exercise, satisfying food, lots of water and a few treats to be happy. Oh, and lots of attention. Oddly, it is not any different on a physical level for humans.

To become more healthy and fit we're not recommending deprivation, instead we are suggesting that you focus on adding the items you are missing in your diet. For a body to be happy and work well it needs to be well oiled (on the right kind of oil), well fed on the right types of foods, well hydrated and properly exercised. To be happy as well as fit, you need to have satisfying relationships with other people as well as a satisfying internal relationship with yourself. (We discuss this in the chapter, "No, No That's Okay.")

Choice #2: Striving toward a Social Expectation.

Many of us were raised knowing size was an issue for our mothers. Sometimes it was an issue for our fathers and siblings too. But most of all weight was a major issue for those of us who were not born with the *perfect* body.

To make matters worse, the *perfect* body changes in our culture from generation to generation. This is why we can't recommend chasing social expectations. In life it is always best to focus on being the best person you can be by understanding who you are and being the best "you" that you can be. Please reconsider Choice #1.

Why is FAT such a dirty word? How bad is fat really?

It is difficult to even pose these questions in America without bringing up a firestorm of emotions from almost everyone. If we look at what the new studies and health data are telling us, it is clear that the healthiest weights are much more varied than originally thought. It is the thinnest in the studies—people with a BMI of below 23—that have the highest risk factors. This is especially true for people who are fifty years and older.

More studies need to be done to determine if fat in itself is any kind of hazard at all to your health. Most studies to date suggest that weight itself is not a threat to health.

This is a very important idea to wake up to when evaluating health and fitness plans for yourself. You need to correctly evaluate the cost benefit ratio of each plan. Here are some examples of real life choices we hear over and over again. If you really believed that fat was deadly they might make sense:

"I smoke to keep from gaining 20 pounds."

> *Reality check:* Smoking is one of the highest risk factors out there. Smoking has absolutely no place in any kind of health and fitness plan. This may even be an idea floated by tobacco companies. Smoking may reduce your appetite, but at what cost?

"I will try any extreme weight loss plan to lose that last 10 pounds."

> *Reality check:* Weight cycling or yo-yo dieting has been found to create health problems. There is strong evidence that weight cycling makes it more difficult for a body to maintain its optimum weight.

"I will try any weight loss drug to try to take the weight off."

> *Reality check:* Most studies put out by drug companies themselves predict an average weight loss of 3–5 pounds total. Is that worth the risk of a long list of negative side effects? The small print for one new weight-loss drug which promised a 3–5 pound total weight loss states you can expect an oily discharge that is not always controllable! (With allies like that who needs enemas?!)

To be healthier mentally and physically you want to create more love, control, fun and freedom in your life. How do you do that?

Take your focus off of your weight and put an end to deprivation.

Our collective focus on weight and fat is misplaced, however it is unmistakable. When you look at today's newspaper headlines and television news, you quickly get the idea that as few as six or seven extra pounds can take years off your life and most Americans should be expecting to die at a younger age.

Consider this: If the now 70 percent "morbidly obese and overweight" Americans were really at a higher mortality rate why hasn't the life expectancy of the average American plummeted?[9] The answer is that the mortality of the average American actually has nothing to do with America's "fatness."

Dire predictions based on overweight and obesity fears do not seem to be reflected in the actual data collected. It looks like there is a flaw in the "FAT is the enemy" line profiteers have been feeding us. Excuse the food pun!

Let's consider why this "fat is bad" myth is so prevalent. The answer is not simple but there is one major component: money. The diet and fitness industry is a $50 billion dollar a year industry. With that much money at stake, it is very profitable to push the idea that thin is better.

You don't have to take our word for it. The research is there for anyone to evaluate. Go to the scientific trials and look at how these studies were devised and carried out and evaluate the conclusions.[10] What we found was a lot of evidence stating just the opposite of what we expected. Fatness is not linked to death in anything but the most extreme cases.

How To Get More Out Of Your Doctor Visits

Many of us have been embarrassed or chastised by doctors after getting on the scale at our yearly check up. It took the authors years to realize that when a doctor believes that weight in and of itself is unhealthy, it can affect the overall level of the healthcare that a person gets. This prejudice can cause a doctor to miss the real cause of an ailment.

Make sure your doctor's office treats you appropriately. For example, you can have total control over being weighed when it is not appropriate. One of the authors went to the doctor because she had something in her eye. The first thing they asked her to do was get on the scale. She refused by saying "I don't think the thing in my eye weighs that much!"

That anecdote may be funny but it strikes at a deeper issue when it comes to the scale. When you think about it, being weighed at every doctor visit doesn't add much to your health or healthcare. What it does do is cause the patient to feel less empowered and take the focus off of the reason for the visit.

Most doctors' offices weigh you automatically every time. You should be able to easily make an agreement with your healthcare provider that lets you control when you are weighed (like in the instance of a large weight gain or loss).

No matter what your size or weight, prejudice is a double-edged sword. It may lead a doctor to make assumptions about health based on weight, even if you are thin.

 Everyone has prejudices about what fitness looks like, so make sure you know which ones your doctor has.

It is always a good idea to talk to and interview your healthcare professionals so that they understand your personal philosophy toward care (e.g., testing before antibiotics), and your family's health history and genetics. Good doctors are open to sound research and individual differences and choices. It is a smart choice to be in charge of your own health and healthcare. Professionals are hired by you to help—not control—your choices. To make good choices it is best to be informed, so do your own research, ask questions and talk to your friends. That is a good way to find a good doctor too. Interview more than one doctor if need be.

If weight still pulls you down try this:

Weight is not (even when combined with height) a measure of health, so what is it? It is a measurement of the pull of the earth on your body. So if the number bothers you consider this:

How would you feel if you gained a *tod* or lost a few *scruples*? Both of these measurements were commonly used in England when agriculture was the primary reason for measuring anything. The following table shows what 170 pounds is when converted to kilograms, stones, tods, scruples and its equivalent on

NEW WAY TO WEIGH CHART					
	IN KILOGRAMS	IN STONES	POUNDS ON MARS	IN TODS	SCRUPLES
= to lbs.	1 kg = 2.2 lbs.	1 Stone = 14 lbs.	1 Mars lb. = 3 lbs.	1 Tod = 28 lbs	1 Scruple = 1 oz.
Formula	Divide Wt. by 2.2	Divide Wt. by 14	Divide Wt. by 3	Divide Wt. by 28	Wt. x 384
Example Weight (Wt.)					
170	**77.2**	**12**	**56.6**	**6.07**	**65,280**
lbs.	Kilograms	Stone	Mars lbs.	Tods	Scruples
Your Weight (Wt.)	Fill in the blanks below!				
lbs.	Kilograms	Stone	Mars lbs.	Tods	Scruples

the planet Mars. Take a look at the chart and find yourself a more comfortable expression of gravity.

In this chapter we have learned that fat is not part of the fitness equation. New research shows fat and fit people live and die at the same rate as thin and fit people do. The real shocker is: lean and unfit people die at the same rate as fat and unfit people.

Remember, fat in and of itself is not the problem.

For most people the greatest health concern is inactivity, which is the real killer. That is why the focus for this book is fitness. The idea is to create more control, fun and freedom in your life, and to do this we *need* to take the focus off the weight and deprivation and put the focus on areas that will create the most change. We encourage you to use the references in this book to do the research yourself. Like we mentioned earlier, to make good choices it is best to be informed. So do your own research, ask questions and talk to your friends.

Exercise Plan

This week's plan is designed to help focus on good measures of fitness so that you can get the most out of your fitness efforts. Fitness reflects more components of your being than just the physical. We'll ask you to look at emotional and mental strength, flexibility and endurance as well as your current abilities in the physical realm.

"NIBBLING AROUND THE EDGE"
WORKOUT CHART

Day 1	• Make a visual (example: a poster, sign, or collage) of three good measures of fitness and display it somewhere where you can see it every day. (Hint: strength, endurance, & flexibility are all good measures of fitness.) **Do not do any additional exercise today.**
Day 2	• Focus on Flexibility: List three examples of your current flexibility. (Don't just focus on the physical. Include mental and emotional as well.) **Do not do any additional exercise today.**
Day 3	• What do you weigh? Weight measurement is a quantification of the pull of gravity on your body. Fill in the Chart in this chapter and find out how much you weigh on Mars. How many tods do you weigh? When people ask what you weigh, now you can pick an alternate to pounds. **Do not do any additional exercise today.**
Day 4	**REST DAY** **Do not do any exercise today.**
Day 5	• Focus on Strength: List three examples of your current strengths. (Don't just focus on the physical. Include mental and emotional as well.) **Do not do any additional exercise today.**
Day 6	• Take control of being weighed. At the doctor's or any other place, *it's your choice.* If you look at being weighed as anything more than information, take a vacation from being weighed. What other information would you like your Medical Doctor to have? **Do not do any additional exercise today.**
Day 7	• Focus on Endurance: List three examples of you how endure. (Don't just focus on the physical. Include mental and emotional as well.) **Do not do any additional exercise today.**

Chapter Endnotes

[5] You might want to know: Dr. Blair's many awards include a MERIT Award from the National Institutes of Health, an ACSM Honor Award, and a Robert Levy Lecture Award from the American Heart Association. He was the Senior Scientific Editor for the U.S. Surgeon General's Report on Physical Activity and Health (1994-1996). Along with many other scientific endeavors he currently serves as a Senior Assoc. Editor, British Journal of Sports Medicine.

[6] *Journal of the American Medical Association* (JAMA), December 2007

[7] Published May 2007 in *Journal of Public Health*

[8] excerpted from: http://www.merriam-webster.com/dictionary/health

[9] The CDC's own data shows that in 2007 America's average life expectancy rate was at an all time high of 77.4 years up from 75 years in 2004.

[10] At the end of this book we have provided a list of resources for anyone wanting to delve into the research further.

No, No, That's Okay!

Changing The Way You Think

This chapter is about that little voice in your head. The type of comments your little voice makes depends on your relationship with yourself. Does your little voice support you, encourage you and treat you with respect?

If you are like most people, your little voice criticizes, blames, complains, nags, threatens and punishes to try to control your behavior. We call that voice "The Internal Critic."

 The Internal Critic is mostly a thinking error that creates more problems than it solves.

This is an extremely radical idea because there is a prevailing myth that if you don't control your behavior with fear, you might spiral out of control. (Remember that all-you-can-eat buffet in the last chapter?) This myth may have started because fear can almost always motivate.

Fear is also a great attention getter. The media uses it constantly. How does the fear serve as a motivator? By creating stress: a grim picture of reality stresses your adrenal glands and the hormone centers in your body, over stimulating these areas.

When you see that fear creates stress, you start to see that fear motivates at a great price. Using fear as a motivator can eventually cost you your ability to move forward. After years of terrorizing yourself into action you may find that you no longer respond to the same old threats inside your head. When your body becomes desensitized fear can manifest itself in a slow, creeping paralysis.

Another major casualty from using fear as a motivator is that it eats away at your ability to enjoy what you have right now. These outcomes are just too high a price to pay for motivation.

Worry and fear can have a large physical impact on health. Fear only motivates as long as you can keep the fear going, and that means you must live in fear to get anything done.

 You don't have to live in fear. This book gives you tools to make other choices.

 The Internal Critic can be modified to eliminate thinking errors.

Modifying the Inner Critic

The first sections of this week's exercises are focused on modifying the Internal Critic. We focus on stopping the fear, and the criticism and then neutralizing the thinking error. We also work at changing the

Internal Critic into a kind and supportive **Internal Evaluator**. Here's an example of how this can happen:

A young college student decided to try modifying her **Internal Critic** for just one week. She started by monitoring the little voice in her head. Whenever she heard her little voice say something like, "You idiot! Why did you say that?" or "You clumsy oaf!" or "You are so fat!" She purposefully countered, either out loud or in her own head, by saying,

"No, no, that's okay!"

At the end of one week she was faced with her first external challenge at a nice dinner with a group of friends. While speaking to the group with expressive hand motions, she accidentally knocked over a beverage. The owner of the spilled beverage blurted out, "I can't believe how clumsy you are!"

The young woman countered without missing a beat,

"No, no, that's okay, I will get you a new beverage."

The blaming student instantly changed his annoyed attitude to one of acceptance because the woman was so self-assured.

Most importantly, the woman reported that even if the other student hadn't been so accepting she would have been okay with the situation. After all it was just an accident. She took responsibility for it and there was no need to place blame.

This experience is an example of how you can work toward changing your experiences and relationships by re-training your **Internal Critic.**

People may think that the **Internal Critic** is like your conscience, helping you distinguish right from wrong, but it is not. Your conscience exists separately, gathering up the information you choose to feed it.

When your conscience gets information from a harsh **Internal Critic,** your response tends to come from a more reactive place.

Your conscience gets better and more accurate information from a calm **Internal Evaluator,** making it easier to distinguish right from wrong.

Be assured, if you cultivate a respectful and loving relationship with yourself by changing your **Internal Critic** into a supportive and loving **Internal Evaluator,** you will find that respectful and loving external relationships become more available.

Now, how does all this relate to fitness? The **Internal Critic** can make it more difficult to find and follow a fitness plan that you can start and, more importantly, stick with.

The **Internal Critic** can make it difficult to properly evaluate your true progress. The more critical the internal voice gets, the less likely you are to step back and honestly evaluate events and goals in your life.

A good example of a very strong **Internal Critic** is someone with anorexia. No matter how thin an anorexic gets, they never feel thin enough. Most anorexics continue to see themselves as fat when they are not. In this extreme case, the thinking error can turn deadly.

The **Internal Critic** gets stronger with years of failed diet and exercise programs. When you are willing to start facing the **Internal Critic** you can move away from living in fear.

One thing that fuels the **Internal Critic** is what you believe will come with fitness. What do you believe fitness brings with it?

- *Celebrity?*
- *Love?*
- *Your own Reality TV show?*
- *Perfect weight control?*
- *A healthier body?*

If you said a healthier body you would be right. The other items on the list are not what you can realistically expect by becoming more fit. It's not that we think you can't have the other items—in fact we believe you can have most of them—but you will have to take actions in other areas beside fitness.

 Give your Internal Evaluator an appropriate fitness focus.

A healthier body is an appropriate fitness focus. Make your goal fitness instead of focusing on body size. You will become healthier mentally and physically, and be able to enjoy the other aspects of your life more readily.

There is an old Native American folktale that applies here:

The Tale Of Two Wolves

A grandmother was talking with her granddaughter.

"A fight is going on inside me," she said to the girl. "It is a terrible fight between two wolves."

"One wolf is angry, envious, war mongering, greedy, full of self-pity, sorrow, regret, guilt, resentment, inferiority, lies, false pride, superiority, selfishness and arrogance."

"The other wolf is friendly, joyful, peaceful, loving, hopeful, serene, humble, kind, benevolent, just, fair, empathetic, generous, true, compassionate, grateful, and is a deep thinker."

"This same fight is going on inside you, and everyone else."

The granddaughter paused in reflection because of what her grandmother had said.

Then she finally cried out, "Grandmother, which wolf will win?"

The wise elder replied, "The wolf that you feed my child...the wolf that you feed."

We'll elaborate on these wolves as a way to illustrate the internal struggle.

The **Internal Critic Wolf:** criticizes, blames, complains, nags, threatens, punishes and bribes inside your head to try to control your behavior. It uses fear to motivate. It lowers self-esteem, and it creates a great deal of stress and worry.

Internal Evaluator Wolf: supports, encourages, listens, accepts, trusts, is respectful and negotiates differences.

Eliminating Thinking Errors

How do you feed the **Internal Evaluator** and pry the **Internal Critic** from your jugular vein? Developing a better relationship with yourself is essential to healthfully reaching your fitness goals. When building a good relationship with yourself, one major thing that can get in your way is wondering what other people think of you. This is different from determining what is right and wrong. It is about the voice that holds you back by saying, "I wish I could do that, but what would 'they' think of me?"

 What others think of you is none of your business.

Thinking about what others are thinking about you is a thinking error (it also feeds the **Internal Critic**). It creates fear to control your behavior and cannot be accurate. It is a waste of time, but more importantly, it can lead to the type of paralysis that stops you from moving forward.

53

If you are thinking about what others are thinking about you, all you need to do is decide to stop. When you notice this thinking error again, decide to stop again and change the focus of your mind. After some practice you will experience a sense of freedom that will grow with even more practice.

Another major stumbling block to building a good relationship with yourself can be the desire to put other people's needs before your own. The desire to care for other people is good, but caring for others and excluding your own needs makes it difficult to show real care for other people. It can also interfere with building a strong **Internal Evaluator**.

Next time you travel on a plane watch the flight attendants; they give out free universal wisdom with the spiel on how to deal with the loss of cabin pressure. You are told to put the oxygen mask on yourself first, *before* trying to help someone else.

Think this through for a minute, why do airlines give these instructions? They give those instructions for a reason. The reason is to counteract the perception that you should help someone else first. In a dire situation like loss of air pressure, if you give in to the urge to help someone else first you will most likely pass out and be unable to help anyone.

 Taking care of yourself first, both mentally and physically, prepares you to take care of others.

When you take care of yourself on a regular basis you provide a good model for the people you care about. Let's face it, the goal for those we care about is not to make them totally dependent on us but to help them find ways to consistently and successfully care for themselves.

Given new information and a feeling of personal power, people improve on the decisions they make, and then they can move forward toward their goals. When you are able to break free from your own fears, you are able to reframe your goals so they become attainable. Insight into your inner self goes a long way.

We think the following piece of prose written by Marianne Williamson (but often misattributed to Nelson Mandela) illustrates our point quite eloquently.

"Our Deepest Fear"
by Marianne Williamson

"Our deepest fear is not that we are inadequate. Our deepest fear is that we are powerful beyond measure. It is our light, not our darkness that most frightens us. We ask ourselves, who am I to be brilliant, gorgeous, talented, fabulous? Actually, who are you *not* to be?"

"... Your playing small does not serve the world. There is nothing enlightened about shrinking so that other people won't feel insecure around you. We are all meant to shine, as children do. We were born to make manifest the glory that is within us. It's not just in some of us; it's in everyone. And as we let our own light shine, we unconsciously give other people permission to do the same. As we are liberated from our own fear, our presence automatically liberates others."

Excerpted from: A Return To Love: Reflections on the Principles of A Course in Miracles[11]

Exercise Plan

This week's exercise plan is designed to help eliminate a thinking error that can interfere with your ability to achieve the goals you set for yourself. By practicing these exercises, it will become easier to envision being more active and empowered.

Chapter Endnotes
_____

[11] *A Return to Love: Reflections on the Principles of A Course in Miracles* by Marianne Williamson © 1992 (Paperback ; pp190-191)

"NO, NO, THAT'S OK" WORKOUT CHART

Day 1	• Stop the Internal Critic. Pay attention to your internal thoughts and say inside your head or even out loud, "No, No, That's OK" each time you catch yourself criticizing yourself during the next week. **Do not do any additional exercise today.**
Day 2	• Read the poem, "Our Deepest Fear", out loud and with feeling! • Continue with exercise from Day One, "No, No, That's OK" **Do not do any additional exercise today.**
Day 3	• List three examples of how you encourage people. Now think of one way you encourage yourself. • Continue with exercise from Day One, "No, No, That's OK". **Do not do any additional exercise today.**
Day 4	**REST DAY** **Do not do any exercise today.**
Day 5	• Take one physical activity that you like to do from the first chapter. • Come up with a list of three reasons you like this activity. (Example; Biking: I like the feel of the road, the wind in my hair, etc.) • Continue with exercise from Day One, "No, No, That's OK". **Do not do any additional exercise today.**
Day 6	• Repeat Day Five's exercise for 10 minutes. Focus on the fun of it. • Continue with exercise from Day One, "No, No, That's OK". **Do not do any additional exercise today.**
Day 7	• Think about the activity you did yesterday for Day Six. Are there other reasons you like doing this activity? • Continue with exercise from Day One, "No, No, That's OK". **Do not do any additional exercise today.**

Using Your Heart to Change Your Mind About Fitness
How Biofeedback Helps You on the Road to Fitness

We've found that one of the best tools for our **Internal Evaluators** is the information provided through Heart Zones™ training, a tool developed by Sally Edwards (see p. 63). Heart Zones™ training uses a heart rate monitor to give you data about your body: this data is known as biofeedback. This biofeedback will give your **Internal Evaluator** lots of accurate information on your current fitness level and your progress toward your goals. This chapter will show the ins and outs of how to use this tool.

Here's a quick example that illustrates the benefit of using biofeedback:

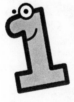 Person #1: She's been "On the Couch" for long enough that she feels very unfit. Walking up stairs really makes her huff and puff. She decides to get in shape and goes out to the local walking path. She remembers when she could run the whole length but decides to walk at a fast clip as a way to ease back in.

Her **Internal Evaluator** tries hard to override the **Internal Critic** who is harping on her to go faster and adds, "This will never work if you don't push harder." For added motivation her **Internal Critic** starts comparing her to the other people on the walking path. Meanwhile, it is physically hard and one of her legs begins to hurt. At the end of her workout she is discouraged and not sure what to do next. And her leg still hurts!

 Person #2: It's the same scenario only she has a heart rate monitor and is using it along with Heart Zones™ training. She heads out to the same path and knows exactly what she wants to do. She watches the biofeedback that she gets from her heart rate monitor and works to stay at the heart rate that she has set for this workout. The **Internal Evaluator** can focus clearly on evaluating what she is doing in line with her specific goals. The **Internal Critic** isn't likely to be silent but when faced with clear evidence of her success the **Internal Critic** fades much more easily into the background. At the end of her workout she feels great and knows exactly when and what she will do next.

 Use information from your heart rate monitor (biofeedback) to silence your Internal Critic and empower your Internal Evaluator.

The above scenarios show the difference between just trying hard without any clear way of knowing what your body is doing versus having and using good biofeedback

Why You Need a Heart Rate Monitor

To get good biofeedback you need a heart rate monitor. You might be thinking, "Not another gadget, to join the other gadgets in the junk drawer." You are right there. There are many heart rate monitors languishing in junk drawers all over the world. The reason for this is that people bought them without learning to use them.

Here is what a typical heart rate monitor looks like:

1.

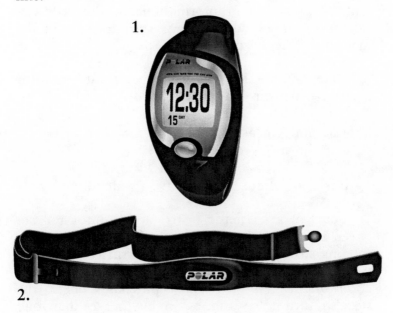

2.

1. *The Monitor:* Looks like (and usually is) a wrist-watch.

2. *The Transmitter Band:* Goes around your chest, right under your bra strap if you're a woman or

under your nipple line if you are a man. The band picks up on the electrical activity of your heart and transmits it to the wrist unit, which shows you the times per minute that your heart is beating. It's pretty cool: you can actually watch your heartbeat!

Tips for Buying a Heart Rate Monitor

If you enjoy the "hunt" and want to checkout websites and compare features, etc., go for it. You will get a lot of good information. But this little section is for those whose heads start to ache at the mention of the word "features."

Here are the features your heart rate monitor needs in order for you to get started:

- It must measure your heart rate.
- It must fit you.

It is also helpful for it to have a watch function.

You can get a basic heart rate monitor for between $40 and $100. These are sold at bicycle stores, running stores, outdoors stores and many outlets on the web. Personally we like Polar, but there are many good brands. As with most purchases check the store's return policy and, before buying, see if anyone there knows how to use the brands they sell.

The New Way to Use the Heart Rate Monitor to Get Fit Faster

The old way to use heart rate information was based on a formula for finding your maximum heart rate, which was 220 minus your age. This formula is wrong and completely outdated. (The old way to use a heart rate monitor included putting it in a drawer for five months before giving it away!)

The new way to use your heart rate depends upon accurately estimating your individual maximum heart rate.

Maximum Heart Rate

Let's talk about maximum heart rate, since it is a key to this training system.

1. What is a maximum heart rate?

Your maximum heart rate is the most beats your heart can beat per minute for any given activity.

2. Why it is it important to know your maximum heart rate?

Because your maximum heart rate is individual to you it can be used to plan a program specifically for you.

3. How do you find your maximum heart rate?

There are two main ways to find your maximum heart rate. One is to do a supervised test and stress your heart in an activity until it cannot beat any faster. The other is to estimate your maximum heart rate using tests that only stress your heart a little.

4. *Does maximum heart rate change as you age?*

No, your maximum heart rate is determined by your individual genetics and is yours for life. What does vary is your ability to get to your maximum heart rate.

 Your maximum heart rate is determined by your individual physiology and genetics and is yours for life.

First Things First

Here comes the part where we remind you to check with your health provider before you start any new workout programs. This is so you understand any limitations you might have. You might be thinking, "Yeah right, blah, blah, blah.... no way am I going to make an appointment to get a lecture from the doctor. I'll wait and go in when I: (pick one)

- Lose weight
- Run a marathon
- Win the Miss Universe pageant

If you thought this, you are not alone. We don't want you to get a lecture from your doctor. We do want you to get some basic information about your specific body. Your **Internal Evaluator** will use this data to correctly evaluate your progress and add to your sense of pride and accomplishment.

Using the attitude and skills mentioned in the earlier chapter on dealing with doctors, we want you to go and get basic information about your blood plus your health provider's okay to start a fitness program. The information about your blood, will help you understand how you process energy, how well your heart is maintaining blood pressure (metabolic health) and if you have any issues that need to be dealt with before you can set forth on this journey.

Here is the data we want you to collect:

1. *Blood pressure:* This can be affected by many things. Having it taken at the beginning and the end of the visit can give you a better sense of your overall blood pressure.

2. *Blood fats (lipids like cholesterol & triglycerides):* Your food intake in the days leading up to this test can affect the outcome. Make sure you follow the doctor's instructions to prepare for the test.

3. *Blood sugar:* There are several kinds of testing scenarios, talk to your doctor about what you should do to prepare.

4. *Hemoglobin levels (especially for women):* This test will let you know if your blood is low in iron (anemia).

Make sure that you understand how to prepare for these tests so you don't influence the results by an accidental triple latte.

This is important: **you do not need to be weighed or measured** unless you really want to be. That is up to you. If your health provider can't hear you, doesn't answer your questions or talks down to you, you have the right and the obligation to find someone who will work with you.

We are <u>NOT</u> suggesting that you ignore concerns your doctor expresses. We are saying that you should be fearless about asking questions, getting second opinions, and researching anything *you* have concerns about, including our recommendations.

Becoming fit may or may not change your weight but is quite likely to change several or all of the other measurements we have listed above.

 The point of having any information is to help you evaluate your progress.

In this way you are going to develop your own u*ser manual* for *your* body.

 You are in charge of your health. Health professionals will be more effective if you can let them know what *you* need to monitor your own health.

Heart Zones™ Training

The Heart Zones™ training system[12] uses your maximum heart rate to calculate "zones." This system is a simple and easy way to get the most out of your heart rate monitor.

The training principles of Heart Zones Training™ are the same for everyone working toward a fitness goal, whether you are Lance Armstrong or someone "Fresh Off the Couch."

Heart Zones Training™, USA was created by Sally Edwards, an accomplished professional athlete and former Master's world record holder in the Ironman™ Triathlon, as well as a world record holder in the Iditashoe 100-Mile Snowshoe Race. Sally has competed in some of the hardest races on the planet, including numerous multi-day adventure races and the Western States 100-Mile Run (which she won). During the 1984 Olympic Marathon Trials she used a heart rate monitor for the first time. Sally combined her master's degree in exercise physiology with her experience as a professional athlete and created the Heart Zones Training System™. Sally is known the world over for her personal success as an endurance athlete; she is also a scientist, author, CEO of Heart Zones™ USA and spokeswoman for the TREK Women's Triathlon series.

Heart Zones™ training uses your maximum heart rate as an "anchor" to provide you with heart rate ranges that are specific to your body.

Estimating Your Maximum Heart Rate

To estimate your maximum heart rate you are going to use tests called submaximum or submax tests. These submax tests keep your heart rate well below your maximum heart rate and are easy to do.

A submax test allows for a good estimate of your maximum heart rate. The results of these tests will give you information to begin to use the Heart Zones™ Training system.

The two submax tests below can be used to predict your maximum heart rate for walking or jogging.

The Chair Test
(Day 5 in the Exercise Plan)

For the *Chair Test* you will need a chair that is easy to stand up from (like a dining room chair), placed on a flat stable surface. You will also need a heart rate monitor and a timer (if the heart rate monitor does not have one).

Wearing your heart rate monitor, sit comfortably and stand up and sit down every three seconds (not fast or slow, just steady). Glance at the heart rate monitor periodically and make a mental note of the rates you see there. At the end, you will want to work with the highest heart rate you saw during the one minute test.

Take that heart rate number and add one of the following Fit Factors to it. (Choose the Fit Factor that best describes your level of exercise over the past month.)

Fit Factors for Chair Test

- **Low**: No daily aerobic physical activity, add **40 beats**

- **Good**: Daily exercise 15 to 30 minutes, add **50 beats**

- **Excellent**: Daily exercise more than 30 minutes most days, add **60 beats**

- **Athlete**: Daily exercise more than 45 minutes most days, add **70 beats**

The Step Test

For the *Step Test* you will need a couple of steps (like indoor stairs) that allow you to step up and down comfortably on a stable, well-lit surface. You will also need a heart rate monitor and timer (if the heart rate monitor does not have one).

For three minutes, step up and down at a comfortable pace. Glance at the heart rate monitor periodically and make a mental note of the rates you see there. At the end, you will want to work with the highest heart rate you saw during the three minute test.

Add one of the following Fit Factors to the results of the *Step Test,* choosing the factor that best describes your level of activity over the past month.

Fit Factors for Step Test

- **Low:** No daily aerobic physical activity, add **55 beats**

- **Good:** Daily exercise 15 to 30 minutes, add **65 beats**

- **Excellent:** Daily exercise more than 30 minutes most days, add **75 beats**

- **Athlete:** Daily exercise more than 45 minutes most days, add **85 beats**

Fill in the blanks below: (bpm = beats per minute)

Chair Test _____ highest bpm + Fit Factor = _____

Step Test _____highest bpm + Fit Factor = _____

Add the results of the Step Test and the Chair Test.

Total of Chair Test and Step Test combined = _____

Now divide that total by 2.

Combined Total divided by 2 = _____ bpm. This is your estimated maximum heart rate.

Remember this number and write it in the space below. This number is your Maximum Heart Rate![13]

My Maximum Heart Rate (100%) _____ bpm

How to Find Your Personal Heart Zones

Now that you have your maximum heart rate, it's time to find your personal heart zones.

The following chart is our modified *Heart Zones™ Chart* which emphasizes the first three heart rate zones.

How to Use the Following Chart

1. Look for the number that is closest to your calculated maximum heart rate along the top line.

2. Underneath each maximum heart rate number is a column with five zones.

3. The boxes underneath your maximum heart rate provide a heartbeat range for each zone. The top two zones are faded into the background. These two zones are important, but because they are very intense we won't cover them in this book.

TRAINING MAXIMUM HEART RATE (BEGINNER'S VERSION)

FIND YOUR MAXIMUM HEART RATE HERE

ZONES	% Max HR	MAX 150	MAX 155	MAX 160	MAX 165	MAX 170	MAX 175	MAX 180	MAX 185	MAX 190	MAX 195	MAX 200	MAX 205	MAX 210	MAX 215	MAX 220
MAX 5 DON'T USE THIS ZONE	100%	150	155	160	165	170	175	180	185	190	195	200	205	210	215	220
	90%	135	140	144	149	153	158	162	167	171	176	180	185	189	194	198
4 DON'T USE THIS ZONE	90%	135	140	144	149	153	158	162	167	171	176	180	185	189	194	198
	80%	120	124	128	132	136	140	144	148	152	156	160	164	168	172	176
3 AEROBIC	80%	120	124	128	132	136	140	144	148	152	156	160	164	168	172	176
	70%	105	109	112	116	119	123	126	130	133	137	140	144	147	151	154
2 TEMPERATE	70%	105	109	112	116	119	123	126	130	133	137	140	144	147	151	154
	60%	90	93	96	99	102	105	108	111	114	117	120	123	126	129	132
1 HEALTHY HEART	60%	90	93	96	99	102	105	108	111	114	117	120	123	126	129	132
	50%	75	78	80	83	85	88	90	93	95	98	100	103	105	108	110

The Five Heart Zones:

Zone 1: The Healthy Heart Zone

- Intensity: Feels Easy
- Percent of maximum heart rate: 50 to 60%

Time spent in this heart zone results in measurable metabolic improvement, enhanced self-esteem, improved blood chemistry, and stabilization of body weight.

Zone 2: The Temperate Zone

- Intensity: Feels moderately easy
- Percent of maximum heart rate: 60 to 70%

This heart zone results in improved energy metabolism and increased cardiovascular endurance.

Zone 3: Aerobic Zone

- Intensity: Feels moderate to almost hard
- Percent of maximum heart rate: 70 to 80%

This heart zone results in measurable improvements in your oxygen-carrying or aerobic capacity, and improved muscle power.

Zone 4 and Zone 5

- Intensity: Hard to very, very, very hard!
- Percent of maximum heart rate: 80 to 100%

The only real reason to train in these zones is to improve sports performance, specifically your body's ability to work non-aerobically or to burn fuel without oxygen.

Get in the Zone, by Finding Yours

Use your maximum heart rate to find your zones and you can prioritize your time and effort to get the most out of your workout time. No more trying to "keep up" with some unrealistic time or distance goal.

"Get in Your Personal Zone!" Chart

Heart Zone 1

Your individual heart rate for Heart Zone 1:

Starts at 50% _____

Ends at 60% _____ (Fill this in)
(50% to 60% of your maximum heart rate)

- Also known as: "Healthy Heart Zone"
- Good for: Getting fit, stress reduction and improving health, increasing the health of your blood chemistry.
- Fuel: Your body uses oxygen to mostly burn fat for fuel.

*To find your heart rate for the zone, check back with your "Personal Heart Zones™ Chart"

Heart Zone 2

Your individual heart rate for Heart Zone 2:

Starts at 60% _____

Ends at 70% _____ (Fill this in)
(60% to 70% of your maximum heart rate)

- Also known as: "The Temperate Zone"
- Good for: Staying fit, basic cardio training, improved fat mobilization
- Fuel: Your body uses oxygen to mostly burn fat for fuel; in this zone it also uses small amounts of readily available carbohydrates.

Heart Zone 3

Your individual heart rate for Heart Zone 3:

Starts at 70% _____

Ends at 80% _____ (Fill this in)
(70% to 80% of your maximum heart rate)

- Also known as: "The Aerobic Zone"
- Good for: Getting fitter, improved aerobic capacity and optimal cardio training
- Fuel: Your body uses oxygen to burn fat and uses the same amount of readily available carbohydrates.

With a heart rate monitor and this Heart Zone chart, you can now see how your personal zones benefit you.

Finally, Some Fun with Heart Rate Monitors!

Now you have a good understanding of the most important aspects of your heart: your **Maximum Heart Rate**. You probably will never see your **Maximum Heart Rate** on your heart rate monitor. The number you will see often on your monitor is your **Ambient Heart Rate** The fancy name for the heart rate you see when you are just sitting around. We encourage you to become very familiar with this heart rate.

Resting Heart Rate is the heart rate you have in the morning *before* you get out of bed. **Resting Heart Rate is different than Ambient Heart Rate,** and you should know the difference. Feel free to check it out, but we won't be talking much about it in this book.

That sitting around heart rate or **Ambient Heart Rate** lets you know how different thoughts, activities, emotions and physical conditions affect your heart. One person we know took to wearing her heart rate monitor at work and used it to get coworkers to back off when they were hounding her by watching her heart rate climb! Someone else wore it during meals and noticed how her heart rate increased between each bite.

As you become more fit you will likely see changes in this heart rate. As you become more familiar with the beat of your own heart you may even be able to use that information to know better when you need rest or even a change of scenery.

Watching your heart rate respond to your daily life gives you information on how your heart reacts to stress.

In this chapter we have started to explore some valuable information that will bring you closer to working out more effectively. If you use a heart rate monitor with your personal heart zones, you provide your **Internal Evaluator** with important information that allows you to quiet your **Internal Critic.** Learning to keep your heart rate in specific zones can move you on the path toward fitness much faster.

Exercise Plan

Becoming familiar with your heart can give you more insight into how to more effectively manage stress. The exercises in this chapter will take you through this process baby step by baby step.

Chapter Endnotes

---

[12] Copyright Heart Zones™ USA

[13] a good estimate of your maximum heart rate

"USING YOUR HEART TO CHANGE YOUR MIND ABOUT FITNESS" WORKOUT CHART

Day 1	• Shopping is not buying! Start looking for a Heart Rate monitor. To start with go for simple. Heart rate, time of day, and stop watch. **Do not do any additional exercise today.**
Day 2	• Buy your Heart Rate monitor! **Do not do any additional exercise today.**
Day 3	• Make an appointment with your health professional to get your metabolic measurements as described in the chapter. • Write out your questions before you go to your appointment to help you take control of your healthcare. You do not have to have your tests results to do the exercises. **Do not do any additional exercise today.**
Day 4	**REST DAY** **Do not do any exercise today.**
Day 5	• Submax Tests: 　　Do the Chair Test and record your result. 　　Do the Step Test and record your result. **Do not do any additional exercise today.**
Day 6	• Using the results of your submax tests plus the fitness factors, fill in the blanks in the section "Estimating Your Maximum Heart Rate" 　　Now you have a good guess at your Max. Heart Rate! **Do not do any additional exercise today.**
Day 7	• Using your Maximum Heart Rate fill in the chart "Get in Your Personal Zone!" **Do not do any additional exercise today.**

78

What's in the Bag?
What Button do I Push?

Tricks of the Trade

It may take a little longer to understand these fitness ideas than you thought it would. But don't be discouraged! Whenever you get a chance, recount every little baby step forward. Remember each step forward is another success.

 In fitness, "the sum of the parts definitely outweighs the whole."

 Every little bit you move, moves you in the right   direction.

Your *"Fitness IQ"* can seem very low at first. Especially when you are "Fresh Off the Couch." Maybe you are truly "fitness information impaired" or maybe it's a kind of denial, not really wanting to know about fitness or just a wee bit of both.

Many very intelligent people live inside their heads and in their emotions, thinking little of the physical fitness world. In fact for many of us, exercise has been little more than a punishment for being fat or out of shape.

Finding the Fun

The trick to reconnecting with your physical self is to think back to when you were a kid and the feeling of playing outside with your friends. Physical activity was just a part of having fun. It was a time in life when running around, jumping, climbing and swimming all seemed a part of everyday life. As a child you probably could spend all day in a pool pretending to swim like fish or running as fast as you could, all for the fun of it.

There is fun to fitness and fun to each physical activity we do. At the risk of sounding like a wacky English nanny, "you find the fun and snap, the job's a game."

Finding the fun in having a physical body, being fit and physical, playing again, is as easy as recalling fun activities we did as children. For example, skipping can still be fun. Just think of what was the most fun in the past: that will be a good place to start for the present. Fun is the key to reconnecting to our physical self. It may also be a slow process, but once you're reconnected to a sense of playfulness, living becomes much more fun and active.

This is the kind of "fitness" that this book is striving to support: enjoying your physical body, finding its strengths and capitalizing on them.

 Fitness should be in service to your life, not the other way around.

Never again will exercise be a punishment for the fat or unfit.

Planning Ahead

 A little planning ahead will make this "fitness thing" a lot easier.

Just like packing your lunch the night before, packing a bag for exercise goes a long way toward helping you get out the door. We recommend packing a bag with everything you need for exercise, so you won't have to go searching for things.

There's not a lot to gather, but imagine having to look for your toothbrush and toothpaste each time you wanted to brush your teeth.

"Oh, no. I left my toothbrush in my other purse!"

"Hmmmm, I think there was some toothpaste in the glove compartment of my car."

"Honey, have you seen the mouthwash?"

"I give up, I'm flossed."

You can see how lack of the right equipment, accessible and ready to go at a moment's notice, might impair a daily routine like teeth brushing or exercise.

We've already talked about buying your heart rate monitor so get a **bag** that can be dedicated to your workout program and put the heart rate monitor in it.

What's in the Bag?

- **Heart rate monitor:** You should have one at this point. Remember to put both parts in the bag.

- **Shoes:** Be sure to get a shoe that fits you correctly and addresses your workout needs. The correct shoe has been known to make exercise comfortable for people with previous breaks or current aches. Find a specialty shoe store that has a liberal return policy. (One of our favorite places is "Super Jock & Jill" in Seattle). Most importantly: get the right size and fit.

   If you have image problems with your feet please consider this: Feet are not too big, too small, too narrow, etc., they are just feet. Shoes on the other hand can be all those things. This is a place to spend money, if you have to. Shoes are very important. So take your time and ask questions.

- **Workout clothes:** Start with one comfortable and attractive outfit for your bag. Why not just wear your old painting clothes? Well, the answer to that is "If you look good... you feel good." That is important because exercise is all about feeling good.

Find an outfit that is <u>not</u> cotton. What else is there, you might ask? Science is a wonderful thing and there are new materials made to wick away moisture from sweat or rain or any soggy combination of the two. It's the material's ability to keep moisture from your body that protects your body temperature. When cotton gets wet it doesn't dry quickly and that can cause your body's core temperature to drop. Being "Fresh Off the Couch" you might sweat less at first but as you get more fit your body will sweat more readily.

- **Socks:** Special socks? That's right, socks are important too. Make sure you have socks that are <u>not</u> made of cotton and that fit well in your workout shoes.

- **Water bottle:** It's always good to have water. When you exercise it's important to stay hydrated. Dehydration can cause problems, so drink water.

What Button Do I Push?

Let's just face it, some of us are more technology oriented than others. Any new technology can be elusive at first. We all have relatives who could never set the clock on the microwave to the correct time. To some, heart rate monitors can seem confusing in the beginning, until you get used to them. Here are some tips:

 I can't get a heart rate on my watch (receiver)!

- Make sure you are pushing the right button to get a heart rate. Check the manual that comes with the heart rate monitor.
- Check your band (transmitter) to make sure it's tight enough around your chest.
- Make sure the band is a little bit wet. Water or sweat conducts the heart rate signal better than dry skin.
- Both parts of the heart rate monitor have batteries; sometimes the batteries can be weak or dead.

If these tips don't help, check with the retailer. If it's been a while since you bought it, check with the company that makes your heart rate monitor for nearby service centers.

Why am I doing all this?

Studies appear daily in the news saying exercise and fitness is "the thing." Weight should not be the focus. Fitness needs to be.

Let's go back to the dog analogy. You know your dog needs a walk every day to be healthy. Being fit is like that for people too. Lifetime habits take time and small baby-step size goals are the way to achieve change. That is what this book is about. It's truly a how-to book on making life changes toward fitness.

In the next chapter we will talk about how to set goals that will lead to real fitness, characterized by flexibility, strength and endurance. Finally we can really take advantage of a positive shift in collective thinking. Instead of growing older and becoming more sedentary, we now see that even as we get older, we can become more fit and more active.

Exercise Plan

This week the plan involves gathering and using all the tools you need to be successful.

"WHAT'S IN THE BAG? WHICH BUTTON DO I PUSH?" WORKOUT CHART

Day 1	• Find a bag that will be dedicated to Working Out. The trick is to fill it with everything you need and keep it ready to go.
	• Here's a basic list of what you will need in your bag:
	    1. Heart Rate Monitor
	    2. Sport Shoes
	    3. Workout clothes
	    4. Water bottle
	      Do not do any additional exercise today.

Day 2	• Identify local sport shoes stores with liberal return policy to insure you get a great shoe for you. **Do not do any additional exercise today.**
Day 3	• Go to sport shoes store and try on shoes. Make sure you can return the shoes if they aren't comfortable. • Buy shoes. Don't forget the socks! **Do not do any additional exercise today.**
Day 4	**REST DAY** **Do not do any exercise today.**
Day 5	• Shop for and purchase appropriate and attractive workout clothes. If you feel attractive you will look attractive no matter what you are wearing. • Look for attractive work out shirts and pants. (Those of us that need larger sizes should look at Target, Brooks and Danskin. Many new companies now cater to larger sizes.) **Do not do any additional exercise today.**
Day 6	• Gather all your new purchases and put them in your dedicated workout bag. Having a bag that is ready to go is half the effort! Now you are all ready to go at a moment's notice. **Do not do any additional exercise today.**
Day 7	• Tweak the heart rate monitor. Put the heart rate monitor on and make sure the band is tight enough without being too tight. • Turn it on, if you don't get a heart rate the band might not be in the correct placement, it might need to be tighter, or it may need to be wet. • Also important to know is that the band or the watch may need a new battery. • As the last resort, check with the manual. **Do not do any additional exercise today.**

Moving the Bull's Eye
Setting Real Fitness Goals

It is important to replace unrealistic weight and body images with realistic fitness goals.

When first letting go of one type of unrealistic goal it's easy to get caught in the sticky web of setting a new type of unrealistic goal. This is one of the most common problems people encounter when they are "Fresh Off the Couch." It's common to see people on new fitness programs, working too hard, too fast, too soon and often for unrealistic goals.

Real fitness goals are based on who you are (genetically as well as culturally) and what your specific desires are. Real fitness goals are also related to your individual physiology (for example your individual maximum heart rate) and your specific needs.

If you are not going to lose weight or fit into a magic size, why try to get fit? Why be fit at all? Real fitness greatly improves your health. It's fun, and does give you a powerful feeling as it reduces stress.

Becoming more active can introduce you to a lot of great active people and can free you in many ways.

Metabolic health (your body's ability to process and use energy) is greatly improved and managing stress can be much easier. Synapses (the communication between your brain and your muscles) get stronger with use and we actually become reconnected to our bodies. Being able to move your body and use your physical strength is a wonderful feeling.

Back to the Dogs

As you already know, dogs need a walk every day to be healthy. You can also see that although healthy, your dog would not be ready to enter into agility trials or other competitions without additional training. Even if your dog was a champion last year, if you had not continued her training, you would not think of reentering her in this year's competition. If the dog did not do extra training, you would not be shocked that she (although healthy) had lost the edge that extra training provides. Well, this is true for people too.

That's why goals are so important. Say you want to enter an event like a triathlon or you want to start with a goal like improving your daily energy flow and reducing stress. Either of these goals needs a plan. The plan needs to be for a finite amount of time.

As you start thinking about making a workout plan, it is important to remember that if you work out too hard, too fast, too soon, it is all too easy to get injured. And if you are lucky enough to <u>not</u> get injured, it is all too easy to think of exercise as too hard to do. So what does that mean?

It is best to start slow. Start with a workout plan that can be easily done, then add on things that can be done with enjoyment as you get more fit. Think about what can be accomplished simply and most importantly, *what you can sustain over time*. That way it is easier to move forward toward better health. But it's equally important to remember that slow, sustainable and enjoyable progress will result in more fun and freedom in your life.

You might well ask how can a fitness program lead to those kinds of life changes?

 By using the Internal Evaluator and quieting a loud Internal Critic you can start making choices that are not motivated by fear.

This change will allow you to feel more peaceful and free, and it will help you to have more fun in your life. With practice we have seen that all these changes together can lead to a feeling of more control over yourself and that enhances your self-esteem.

Fitness is a moving target that is totally defined by what you want. In fact "fitness" means a lot of different things. For example, a gymnast, a long distance runner or someone who just wants to improve his or her health would have very different workouts. In fact, even the same person would train differently for different goals. Remember, workout plans for those "Fresh Off the Couch" share many important characteristics with workout plans of the most competitive athletes. And like the competitive athlete, those "Fresh Off the Couch" must have a plan that is well inside their ability to achieve.

Traits Successful Workout Plans Have in Common

 Consistency: Consistency achieves the best results.

Based on individual characteristics: (like maximum heart rate) for an "anchor:" Using individual characteristics in your workout plan makes it easier to train effectively.

 Variety and recovery: Including these gets better results in all workout plans.

Consistency can be built more successfully if you are willing to take it slow.

 There is power in starting with achievable goals and measuring the results over time.

You will find that noting small successes over time can be very empowering.

Heart rate monitors are invaluable when it comes to letting you know what your body is doing. Accurate biofeedback allows you to know on a minute-to-minute basis if you are succeeding at the workout you planned. It also allows you to see incremental changes in your improving fitness.

Almost everyone will say that they have a good idea what their heart is doing before they start using a heart rate monitor. That's funny, because when you start using a heart rate monitor as we have described in the last chapter, you will be amazed how far off you can be from what your heart is actually doing.

When using a heart rate monitor for the first time, one woman reported feeling like she was "walking in molasses." She felt her heart pumping hard and her legs heavy as lead, were barely coming off the ground when she walked around the track. When she finally checked her heart rate monitor she found her heart was not beating very fast at all. She was then able, with this input, to shake off her sluggish perception and move her heartbeat up to her target Heart Zone.

The same woman reported having a very easy day of it and was moving fast around the track. When she checked her heart rate monitor this time, it had moved above the heart zone where she wanted to train. She found she had to slow down to keep her heart rate where it should be for her training plan. Her experience is actually quite common. This shows how the immediate biofeedback of the heart rate monitor can help you get so much more from your workout plans.

We have developed a starting plan for you, but you will have to come up with the goal that will take you beyond the scope of this book. Here are two types of fitness goals to start thinking about:

"Process" Goals (a.k.a., doing goals) – Examples: "I'm going to walk ten minutes in Heart Zone 3 three times a week" or "I'm going to wear my heart rate monitor two hours a day to see how my heart rate varied through out the day."

"Achieving" Goals (a.k.a, end point goals) – Examples: "I want to be able to walk around the block comfortably in Heart Zone 3 without stopping" or "I

want to comfortably finish a 5K walking event for charity."

Process goals and achieving goals often work together. The key to success is making sure that they are a fit for you. There are a couple of things that will be true of any plan that we are advocating here:

- We are only using your first three heart zones (50 percent to 80 percent of your maximum heart rate).
- Every plan will strive for each workout to feel "really easy." As you become more fit you will have to adjust your plan to better suit your desires and your goals.

 Rest is as important as the workout. Truly taking a break from what you are doing can actually result in big steps forward in progress.

It is a mistake for those starting out to think that because what they are doing doesn't seem like much, they do not need rest from it. It is true that many starting out will not strictly need a rest from a light workout, but there is more to "rest" than just the physical stress that you put on your body. There is "rest" from having to find time away from other activities and mental "rest" from getting yourself ready. As you progress, "rest" and "recovery" will be crucial to moving forward toward your fitness goals whatever they might be.

Planning and limiting your workouts to a specific goal on both time and intensity will lead to big steps forward in your fitness progress.

As you already know, you don't have to workout as hard as you can as often as you can. So what do you do instead? Set the length and intensity of your workout to get the most out of your workout in the shortest amount of time.

Using the Internal Evaluator With Heart Zones™ to Set Intensity

(Here is how to do the exercises described in the exercise chart for this week)

 Using Heart Zone 1 pick any activity that you can do comfortably, (for this example we will use walking) and start your heart rate monitor. Aim to keep your heart rate in Heart Zone 1 for ten minutes.

Answer these questions:

1. Could you stay in Heart Zone 1 without stopping your activity?

   This zone is low intensity so do not be surprised if you had to stop and start to keep your heart rate in Heart Zone 1— *that is pretty normal.*

2. Could you breathe and talk in Heart Zone 1?

   If you weren't able to breathe comfortably and talk it could mean that your maximum heart rate is set too high in which case redo the Chair and Step Tests in Chapter 4. If you think the results were accurate, this is really important information because now you know that your heart needs to work in this zone for a while so it can get stronger.

3. Did you feel like you could do the activity longer?

   If you felt you could do the activity easily for longer that is good! If it felt like a challenge, that's good too, because you now know to start with ten minutes.

4. Did you feel comfortable?

   This is a tricky question because you might be feeling awkward or vulnerable trying new things; this kind of discomfort is normal and part of the process. However pain is not and should be addressed. Sometimes when people move from being unfit to more fit they are embarrassed. Sometimes they think that pain is just part of the process. It is not. If the shoes cause pain do not hesitate to go back to the store and get them to help you figure it out. If you experience joint pain or any other physical pain do not hesitate to get examined by your health professional.

 If you have decided that you should start your work out in **Heart Zone 1:**

- Work out in this zone only for 10 to 20 minutes.

If Heart Zone 1 was easy, repeat the ten minutes in Heart Zone 2 and then answer the questions from pages 93-94.

 If you have decided that you should start in **Heart Zone 2:**

- Work out in this zone only for 10 to 20 minutes.
- Warm-up in Heart Zone 1 for two minutes. Cool down after your workout in Heart Zone 1 for two minutes.

If Heart Zone 2 was comfortable and felt easy you can go on to trying Heart Zone 3.

If you just did the first two zones you will be warmed up. If not, spend about two minutes in Heart Zone 2 warming up. Then increase your activity slowly and note how you feel.

 If you have decided that you should start your workout in **Heart Zone 3:**

- Work out in this zone only for 10 to 20 minutes.
- Warm-up in Heart Zone 1 or 2 for two minutes.
- Cool down after your workout in Heart Zone 1 or 2 for two minutes.

The exercises above let you determine what intensity will get you the best results in the fastest time. Starting at a level that is <u>too hard</u> will not get you fit faster.

The focus has to be on what will be sustainable over time.

Fun Fact: When your body is stressed aerobically (meaning you are in that "still able to talk" mode) the muscles signal the body to make more mitochondria (cells within our body that have separate DNA). Mitochondria are the fat burning energy production factories when there is enough oxygen available.

Workout Plan Basics

Let's review the basics to creating your own workout plan:

1. Remember it's like brushing your teeth or like walking your dog; a work out plan needs to be consistent and regular.

2. Using the exercises above to set the length and intensity of your workout will allow you to customize your workout so you can train smarter and more efficiently with better results because they are geared to you as an individual.

3. Every plan should also include rest and recovery.

4. Every training session should include a warm up and cool down because they are not just physical transitions; they are mental transitions too.

 ## Pre-flight Check (Warm-up)

During the warm up you should focus on your goals for the training and do a little "pre-flight" check on your body. Notice how you're moving and how everything feels. As pointed out earlier some discomfort is fine but pain is not. Also notice the conditions you are working out in. Is it hot? Will you need water? Too dark? Too cold? Do you have the right clothes? How is your body responding?

 ## Post-flight Check (Cool-down)

In cool down, do a "post-flight" check and let your heart rate return to an easy comfortable level before you end your workout. Don't worry if your warm up and cool down start out feeling pretty awkward, they will improve as you do!

In case you need some 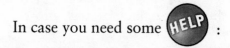 :

All this technical stuff can feel overwhelming, but don't worry. This week's workout program will incorporate all these new ideas and you can follow it until you are ready to move on to something new. As you become more comfortable with the ideas in this book (which are actually *Radical* and take some practice to get used to), you will be able to come back and incorporate sections that you skipped over in the beginning. This is fine, as long as you keep moving and use the heart rate monitor for accurate biofeedback.

 Real evidence of your increased fitness turns into real motivation, free of fear. And that is real power!

Exercise Plan

This week's plan will help you to understand and set real fitness goals. No matter what intensity level you start to work out in, you will find as your fitness increases you will need more activity to raise your heart rate to get into the zone you picked.

"MOVING THE BULL'S-EYE" WORKOUT CHART

Day 1	• List three goals you have accomplished. • Identify if the goals were Process Goals, Achieving Goals or a combination of the two. (These don't have to be fitness goals.) **Do not do any additional exercise today.**
Day 2	• Spend 10 minutes in your Heart Zone 1. • Answer the questions in section "Using The Internal Evaluator with Heart Zones to Set Intensity" in this chapter. **Do not do any additional exercise today.**
Day 3	• Spend 10 minutes in your Heart Zone 2. • Answer the questions in section "Using The Internal Evaluator with Heart Zones to Set Intensity" in this chapter. **Do not do any additional exercise today.**
Day 4	**REST DAY** **Do not do any exercise today.**
Day 5	• Spend 10 minutes in your Heart Zone 3. • Answer the questions in section "Using The Internal Evaluator with Heart Zones to Set Intensity" in this chapter. **Do not do any additional exercise today.**
Day 6	• Practice your Pre-flight Check (Warm-up) for 2 minutes. Pay attention to how your clothes and shoes and heart rate monitor feel. • Using the intensity of heart zone you are comfortable at exercise for 10 minutes. • Practice your Post-flight Check (Cool-down) for 2 minutes. Take note of your heart rate and how your body feels. **Do not do any additional exercise today.**
Day 7	• Warm-up for 2 minutes. • Pick two heart zones that you are comfortable in. For 10 minutes move back and forth between the two heart zones. • Cool-down for 2 minutes. Take note of your heart rate and how your body feels. **Do not do any additional exercise today.**

99

Moving Forward

Start Living Now

Comedian Louie Anderson, in one of his well-loved routines, talks about getting advice from his drunken father. Louie imitates his dad trying to pass on the wisdom of the ages with intoxicated urgency, "Louie," his dad would say, "Life... Live it!" It seems like pretty minimal advice, so goes the joke, but it is good advice to those of us who have put our lives on hold because we want to be thinner, weightier, richer, prettier, and healthier before we start living. The ideas in this book are to help you start living now!

 Start living now, and get more of what you want.

Within each chapter we placed weekly exercises designed to increase fun, freedom, power, love and (last, but not least) fitness.

◈ 1 ◈

In "**Begin Where You Are**" we introduced Choice Theory and the radical notion that you are in control of your fitness choices. You learned that gaining mental awareness and taking responsibility for your fitness choices will help you exercise your freedom as well as your physique.

In the same chapter, you read about realistic body types versus the myths put forth by various media. You took a look at your family's gene pool to get in touch with your physical starting point, and to help your perspective, we asked you to think about what breed of dog your body type most resembles and what the AKC standards might be for your individual breed. You also learned a more effective way of starting on the road to fitness: you've begun to look at fitness as a healthy habit, like brushing your teeth. For healthy teeth you need to clean them daily and for a healthy body you need to take up daily exercise. Also in that chapter, you became acquainted with the radical idea that:

 Your fitness routine, like your dental routine, needn't take up lots of time.

Finally, "Begin Where You Are" emphasized that it is important to take the focus off of weight and put it on fitness, where it belongs.

◈2◈

In "Nibbling Around the Edges" we clarified that weight, height and any combination of the two is no measure of health. It is only a measure of your weight and height. You learned to think of those measurements as data and free yourself from fitness judgments based on those numbers. You learned that the BMI is based on a measure of height and weight and, therefore, is not a measure of health or fitness. You learned to replace those outdated and useless measures with valid fitness indicators: strength, flexibility and endurance.

You became aware that assumptions about fitness based on size can cause healthcare professionals to overlook valid fitness indicators, and you learned to challenge those assumptions with questions and data. "You can't be too rich or too thin," is a popular saying, but studies show being too thin actually increases your health risks significantly, especially for people born before or during the baby boom. In "Nibbling Around the Edges" you learned why:

 It is important to take the focus off of weight and put it on fitness where it belongs.

◈3◈

"No, No, That's Okay" is the chapter in which we identified a thinking error that can be the cause of paralysis in the fitness area and the cause of misery in other areas of your life. If self-criticism is too strong it can slow down or stop growth completely. Worse, this thinking error can make it impossible to enjoy what you currently have in your life.

Practicing the weekly exercise plan in "No, No, That's Okay," helps turn the **Internal Critic** into an **Internal Evaluator**. The result is that you are better able to evaluate goals correctly and move forward at a steady clip. More importantly, changing the **Internal Critic** into an **Internal Evaluator** allows you to truly enjoy your progress. These exercises take practice and as you have already learned; practice is not perfection.

Practice is just practice. Steady, regular practice is all that is needed for any of these ideas to be successful.

One impressive study we looked at while researching this book had evidence suggesting another important thing you can do for yourself is to have a positive attitude. The evidence suggested a positive attitude[14] with no other changes would add years to your life. This means that just changing your attitude toward life can have a significant effect on how long you live.

 Eliminating the over-critical thinking error will go a long way toward having more power in your life.

That, in turn, will create more of a positive feeling in your life.

What really counts is realizing that: you and you alone have control over yourself.

 When you realize you are the only one who can change yourself, that's where your power begins.

So many people get stuck on the nowhere loop of trying to change others or blaming others for their situation. Remember Christopher Reeves: It was not his choice to be in a wheelchair, but definitely his choice to live his life fully.

◈4◈

Learning how to incorporate biofeedback into your fitness plan is important information that was covered in "Using **Your Heart to Change Your Mind About Fitness.**" Fitness research over the last twenty years has changed the way we think about how the body works. A significant change--beside the way we now think about weight--is how to use a heart rate monitor to gain endurance faster and more effectively. Within this chapter you learned an easy way to estimate your Maximum Heart Rate and how to use Heart Zone Training™ to make your exercise more fun and effective.

You learned that your Maximum Heart Rate is yours for life, and that using age to calculate maximum heart rate is another outdated and useless idea. In "Using Your Heart..." you found evidence that:

 You can be fit or unfit at any age, just like at any weight or height.

Now that you have read most of this book we bet you could have guessed that!

 No longer focusing on diets frees up time and energy to achieve your real goals.

A thin body will not bring fitness, power, love and belonging. If thinness will not give you these things, what will? Just realizing this gets you closer to your real goals.

In **"What's in the Bag? What Button do I Push?,"** we went over what you will need to have on hand to simplify the transition from couch person to active person.

 Having items in the bag and ready to go actually makes being active possible.

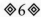

The chapter **"Moving the Bulls' Eye"** discussed how to set real fitness goals. When you realize what fitness is, you can better set goals that increase your strength, flexibility and endurance. The false belief that low weight equals good fitness can make it impossible to set real fitness goals. Resetting the measures of good health frees you to set reasonable goals that will improve your actual fitness.

 When you focus on attainable goals, you can actually achieve them. That means big goals are best achieved in baby steps.

◈7◈

If we are able to convey only one idea in this book let it be that pursuing fitness should be in service to your life. Avoid shaming yourself into becoming more fit. Instead, pursue fitness because fitness makes a physical life on this planet more fun. And a fit body is more energetic and more enjoyable to have.

Exercise Plan

This exercise plan provides you with a basic workout that if used over time, will move you toward sustainable fitness.

Chapter Endnotes
_____

[14] Levy BR, et al. Longevity increased by positive self-perceptions of aging. *Journal of Personality and Social Psychology*. 2002 Aug; 83(2): 261-70.

"MOVING FORWARD" WORKOUT CHART

Day 1	**Heart Zone 2 Workout** • Warm-up for 2 minutes. • Maintain your Heart Rate in Heart Zone 2 for 10 to 20 minutes. • Cool-down for 2 minutes. **Do not do any additional exercise today.**
Day 2	**Heart Zone 3 Workout** • Warm-up for 2 minutes. • Maintain your Heart Rate in Heart Zone 3 for 10 to 20 minutes. • Cool-down for 2 minutes. **Do not do any additional exercise today.**
Day 3	**Interval Heart Zone Workout** • Warm-up for 2 minutes. • Start at the lowest heart rate in Heart Zone 2 for 1 minute. • Go to the middle of Heart Zone 3 for 1 minute. • Repeat for a total of 10 to 20 minutes. Cool-down for 2 minutes. **Do not do any additional exercise today.**
Day 4	**REST DAY** **Do not do any exercise today.**
Day 5	**Heart Zone 2 Workout** • Warm-up for 2 minutes. • Maintain your Heart Rate in Heart Zone 2 for 10 to 20 minutes. • Cool-down for 2 minutes. **Do not do any additional exercise today.**
Day 6	**Heart Zone 3 Workout** • Warm-up for 2 minutes. • Maintain your Heart Rate in Heart Zone 3 for 10 to 20 minutes. • Cool-down for 2 minutes. **Do not do any additional exercise today.**
Day 7	**Interval Heart Zone Workout** • Warm-up for 2 minutes. • Start at the lowest heart rate in Heart Zone 2 for 1 minute. • Go to the middle of Heart Zone 3 for 1 minute. • Repeat for a total of 10 to 20 minutes. Cool-down for 2 minutes. **Do not do any additional exercise today.**

Recommended Reading

Obesity Myth by Paul Campos

Heart Zone Training by Sally Edwards

Big Fat Lies by Glenn A. Gaesser

Obesity Epidemic: Science, Morality and Ideology by Michael Gard and Jan Wright

Rethinking Thin by Gina Kolata

Fat Politics by Eric Oliver

We'd love to hear from you!

Please visit our website:

www.freshoffthecouch.com

About the Authors

Cris Kessler has a MSW from the University of Washington. She is a Heart Zones™ Level III Coach and Personal Trainer, Adjunct Faculty of the Graduate School of Social Work, University of Washington, Seattle; Faculty William Glasser Institute. Cris has been a Social Worker for over twenty-five years and a Heart Zone Trainer for the past five years. Cris is happily married and lives in Seattle with her family. She has raced in triathlons for the last twelve years, finishing in the top three in her weight and age class for both Olympic and Half Ironman distances. Cris is co-founder of Cognitive Fitness, a company created to teach those who want to be fit how to use their heart to change their mind about fitness.

Marla Fields has a BS in Psychology from the University of Wisconsin. She has been an Instructor for over ten years, most recently at Lake Washington Technical College. She is a produced writer for television and film. Marla grew up in Madison, Wisconsin but has lived and worked on the west coast for over twenty years. She is happily married and lives with her family in Seattle. Marla is co-founder of Cognitive Fitness, a company created to bring fitness to everyone who wants it, even if they are still on the couch just thinking about getting fit.

Printed in the United States
153163LV00002B/33/P

9 781934 733332